20 TIPS FOR *Success*

1. KEEP A FOOD JOURNAL
Studies have shown that keeping a journal is the most important tool for losing weight and keeping it off. It's also been proven that the simple awareness of exactly what you eat could in itself reduce body weight.

2. COUNT CALORIES
More important than anything else, you want to control calories while trying to lose weight, so be sure to keep track of how much you're taking in each day.

3. WEIGH YOURSELF EVERYDAY
A study in the *Annals of Behavioral Medicine* found that it's helpful if you're trying to lose weight, and there's no proof that doing so will depress or discourage you: Research from the University of Minnesota School of Public Health found no strong connection between frequent weigh-ins and depression in women. Also, self-weighing daily was associated with lower Body Mass Index in women **40** and up.

4. USE SMALLER PLATES & UTENSILS
Use smaller plates and smaller utensils — and put down the silverware between bites.

5. EAT SLOWLY
A study at the University of Rhode Island showed that when women shoveled down their food, they consumed far more calories than when they took their time, taking smaller bites and chewing more times before swallowing. They were also less satisfied and hungrier an hour after eating a meal quickly than when they ate slowly.

6. NO DISTRACTIONS
Sit down to eat and don't do anything else— don't read, watch TV, or drive.

7. DON'T GO FOOD-SHOPPING HUNGRY
Be sure to eat something healthy 30 minutes before you go to the store, and you'll be able to resist all those junk-food impulse buys.

8. READ NUTRITION LABELS
Besides calories and fat, avoid foods with high sugar and sodium levels.

9. DON'T DEPRIVE YOURSELF
You should never be hungry. Try eating six smaller nutritious meals a day so you won't be starved.

10. HIDE FOODS THAT MIGHT TEMPT YOU
Put them at the back of the fridge or cupboard, or keep them in a covered dish. Studies have shown you'll eat significantly more food if it's in close proximity or visible.

11. DON'T BRING SERVING DISHES TO THE TABLE
Leave serving dishes on the counter or in the kitchen, so you don't just mindlessly take another helping.

12. BEWARE OF "LOW FAT" FOODS
Foods labeled "low fat" aren't necessarily low in calories. Often there is extra sugar in reduced-fat foods. The body also needs fat to function properly, so you don't want to cut it out of your diet completely.

13. EAT MUSTARD INSTEAD OF MAYO
Other more healthful condiments: salsa, horseradish, and ketchup. Making simple substitutions with similar, often more flavorful but lower-calorie foods can make a big difference.

14. BUY MORE EXPENSIVE/SPECIAL FOODS
If they are special and pricey, chances are you'll eat less of them, and more mindfully.

15. NOTICE WHEN YOU ARE FULL
Stay attuned to internal vs. external hunger cues: feelings of fullness, as opposed to the fact that there's more food on your plate.

16. BE CAREFUL WHAT YOU DRINK
Beverages make up half of the "extra" calories we consume. Water is always best, but if you choose juice, dilute it with water. Try to avoid high-calorie soda: Scientists say the body responds to liquid calories differently than it does to calories from food. You could drink a huge soda with far more calories than a big burger but still feel hungry.

17. BE SURE TO HYDRATE
Drinking too little can prevent you from losing weight, because dehydration can slow your metabolism.

18. HYDRATE FREQUENTLY
It's not how much water you drink, it's how frequently. Sipping small amounts often is better than gulping down full glasses at once.

19. MEN & WOMEN LOSE WEIGHT DIFFERENTLY
It's been proven that men lose more rapidly (most likely due to the fact that women need to maintain more body weight to carry babies). Keep this in mind if you're dieting along with your partner or spouse.

20. DON'T EAT OUT OF JARS OR BAGS
Put food on a plate so you can see what and how much you're eating.

100 CALORIE SERVINGS

Calories do count—keeping track of how many calories you take in is a good way to control your diet. Below, we've listed a variety of one-hundred-calorie food servings that you can use as a guide when you are filling out your food logs.

dairy

1 oz blue cheese

1 oz American cheese *(106)*

1 oz Edam

1 oz Gouda

1 oz provolone

3/4 oz cheddar

1 string cheese stick

1/2 cup egg substitute

1 Tbsp margarine

1 Tbsp mayonnaise

1/2 cup low-fat (2%) cottage cheese

2 Tbsp cream cheese

1/2 cup yogurt w/fruit *(113)*

3 oz fat-free frozen yogurt

1 medium hard-boiled egg *(81)*

veggies

5 cups raw mushrooms

2/3 cup canned peas

2 large sweet gherkins

1 cup boiled potatoes

3 cups cabbage

2 artichokes

2 cups canned asparagus (94)

4 Tbsp raw avocado

1/2 cup lentils (106)

2 cups cooked carrots

3 cups cooked cauliflower

2 cups collard greens

22 large whole green olives

2 cups frozen spinach (94)

4 cups summer squash

2 cups canned tomatoes (96)

20 water chestnuts

45 steamed edamame

fruit

1 medium banana

30 grapes

2 peaches or 1/2 cup canned syrup-packed peaches

1 Bartlett pear

2 cups strawberries (110)

2 cups cantaloupe

20 cherries

1/2 cup cranberry sauce, sweetened

5 dates (108)

2 slices honeydew (1/5 of a melon)

1 cup pineapple tidbits, in water (96)

3 plums

1/2 apple with 2 tsp peanut butter

1 cup mango chunks

1 cup blueberries

2 cups raspberries

2 cups blackberries

meat, fish & poultry

2 oz chicken, light meat, no skin

2 oz fish sticks

2 oz lamb

2 oz lean roast beef

1 oz pork (Boston butt)

2 oz salmon

2 links pork sausage

2 oz turkey, light meat, no skin (90)

2 oz turkey salami

3 oz turkey pastrami

2 slices beef tongue

1 cup fresh cooked crab (106)

4 sardines

3 oz flounder

3 oz lobster

3 oz tuna, white chunk (105)

3 oz sea bass (105)

2 oz scallops

bread & pasta

1 cup Cheerios

1 cup corn flakes

1 cup Wheaties

1 cup cooked farina

1/2 cup cooked granola

1/3 cup Wheat Chex (110)

1 packet instant oatmeal (mixed with water)

8 saltines

1/2 cup egg noodles

1 whole flour tortilla (108)

5 Triscuits

1 Thomas' 100-calorie muffin or bagel

12 mini rice cakes

1 slice French bread

drinks

12-oz can ginger ale (108)

1-oz package cocoa mix

1 cup grapefruit juice

1 cup low-fat (1% or 2%) milk

1/2 cup evaporated milk

1/2 cup prune juice

4 oz table wine

8 oz beer

12 oz Gatorade (90)

2 cups coffee with cream (90)

8 oz orange juice (115)

8 oz root beer and a scoop of non-fat vanilla frozen yogurt (90)

HOW TO BURN 100 CALORIES

20 minutes of bicycling

15 minutes of brisk walking

15 minutes of skipping rope

15 minutes of an aerobics
  video

30 minutes of yoga

15 minutes of jogging

20 minutes of dancing

20 minutes of walking
  briskly up and down
  the stairs

20 minutes of brisk
  housecleaning
  (vacuuming, scrubbing,
  dusting)

25 minutes of ironing

30 minutes of washing
  the car

25 minutes of gardening

30 minutes of raking leaves

15 minutes of swimming

20 minutes of golfing

30 minutes of playing
  Frisbee

35 minutes of pushing
  a baby stroller
  (or two leisurely
  20-minute strolls)

25 minutes of mowing
  the lawn

20 minutes of painting walls

15 minutes of vigorous
  weight-training

15 minutes of
  shoveling snow

25 minutes of Hula-hooping

15 minutes of beach
  volleyball

30 minutes of playing
  with the dog

30 minutes of mopping

Kissing 10 or 11 times

TIPS FOR Eating Out

- Only eat half of what you order. Ask for a doggy bag for the rest before you even begin your meal.

- Order a salad and appetizer instead of an entrée.

- Eat salads and veggies first, then meats and starches. You'll be full enough after eating all the lower-calorie, high-fiber foods that you'll be content with smaller portions of the others.

- Always share dessert. Especially in groups, you can order several sweet choices and just have a bite or two of each.

- Pick foods that are steamed, baked, roasted, broiled, or grilled -- not fried.

- Choose marinara or wine sauces instead of cream, butter, oil or pesto.

- Get sauces and dressings on the side and use them as dips.

- Starting with soup may help you eat less overall. It forces you to eat more slowly, and most kinds are low in fat and calories. Just avoid soups made with cream.

- Avoid buffets and "all you can eat" specials.

- Instead of counting on yourself to eat out healthfully during the workday, brown-bag your lunch.

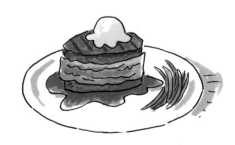

Carrot cake

CARROT CAKE = **415** CALORIES

1 Start with a small carrot.

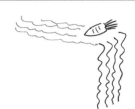

2 Add four squiggly vertical lines...

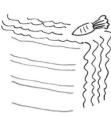

3 ...and four squiggly almost horizontal lines.

4 Draw six barely curved lines.

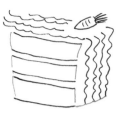

5 Connect the sides and bottom.

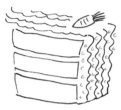

6 Add lots of little c's.

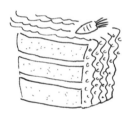

7 Tap lots of dots. The faster you do this, the more calories you will burn.

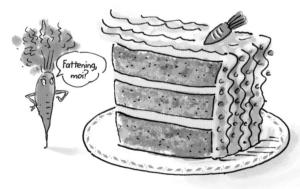

Fattening, moi?

8 Add a plate. The smaller the plate, the bigger your piece of cake will look.

CALORIES EATEN:

_____ _____ _____ _____ _____

appetizer + main + dessert + drinks = total

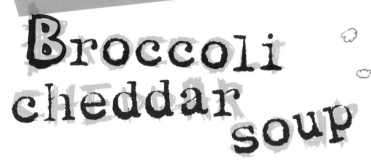

Broccoli cheddar soup

1 Draw seven squiggly blobs of broccoli.

2 Add five slivers of cheese...

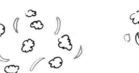

3 and five bits of bacon.

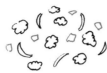

4 Draw two ovals around...

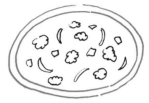

5 one curve inside and one curve outside.

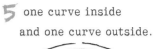

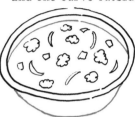

BROCCOLI CHEDDAR SOUP = **407** CALORIES

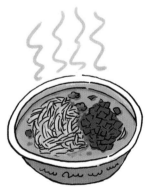

6 Dump in a load of cheese and a load of bacon while it's hot.

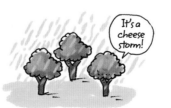

It's a cheese storm!

CALORIES EATEN:

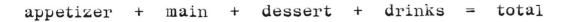

appetizer + main + dessert + drinks = total

Manhattan

MANHATTAN = **210** CALORIES

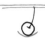

1 Start with a cherry.

2 Add two straight lines on top and a curve on the bottom.

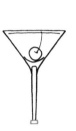

3 Draw a skinny loop.

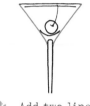

4 Add two lines...

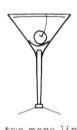

5 a little box...

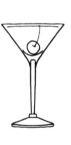

6 two more lines.

7 Attach a loop.

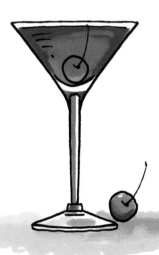

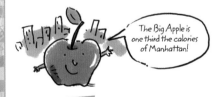

The Big Apple is one third the calories of Manhattan!

CALORIES EATEN:

_____ + _____ + _____ + _____ = _____

appetizer + main + dessert + drinks = total

Apple pie

APPLE PIE = **470** CALORIES

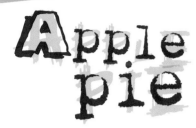

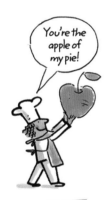

You're the apple of my pie!

appetizer + main + dessert + drinks = total

1   Start with a big scoop of vanilla ice cream.

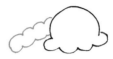 2   Attach a fat squiggle.

3   Draw two squiggly L-shaped lines...

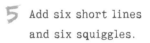 4   and one squiggly V-shaped line.

5   Add six short lines and six squiggles.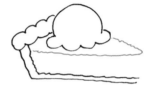

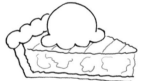 6   Put a smooth oval and a squiggly oval all around.

7   The pies have it.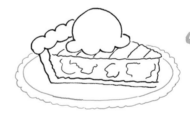

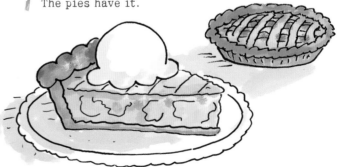

French fries

FRENCH FRIES = **590** CALORIES

1 Draw a curvy V and I.

2 Make them fat.

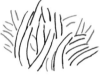

3 Add three pairs of curves...

4 and five more pairs of curves...

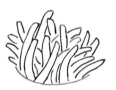

5 and nine more pairs of curves.

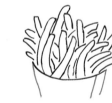

6 Close the top ends of each pair.

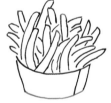

7 Draw one big curve and four small curves.

8 Attach three vertical lines . . .

9 and connect with a big curve.

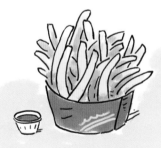

10 And get some catsup.

CALORIES EATEN:

_____ _____ _____ _____ _____

appetizer + main + dessert + drinks = total

Cherry cheesecake

CHERRY CHEESECAKE = **450** CALORIES

1 Draw eight stemless cherries in a row.

2 Add seven small curves above and...

3 a squiggly line below.

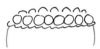

4 Draw two vertical curves on either end...

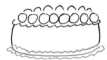

5 and three horizontal curves.

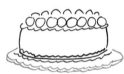

6 Add two more squiggles on the bottom...

7 and two vertical curves on the bottom.

8 Finish with two more squiggles.

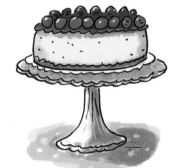

CALORIES EATEN:

___ + ___ + ___ + ___ = ___

appetizer + main + dessert + drinks = total

Everything bagel

EVERYTHING BAGEL = **780** CALORIES

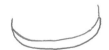

1 Draw two smiling bagel curves.

2 Slather on a squiggly curve of cream cheese...

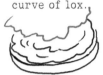

3 and spread it.

4 Add a really squiggly curve of lox...

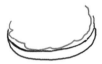

5 Draw two smooth curves and four u's of tomato.

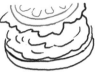

6 Add a really, really squiggly curve of lettuce...

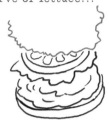

7 and three slivers of red onion.

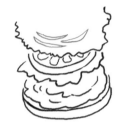

8 Put on the bagel top...

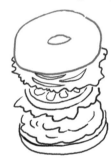

9 and everything on top of that.

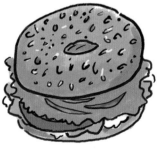

10 Carefully press down so that all of the calories ooze out the sides.

CALORIES EATEN:

_____ _____ _____ _____ _____

appetizer + main + dessert + drinks = total

Wedding cake

WEDDING CAKE = **347** CALORIES

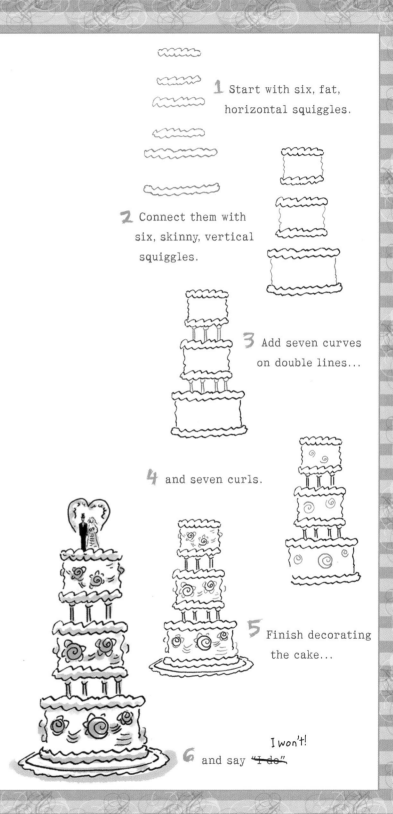

1 Start with six, fat, horizontal squiggles.

2 Connect them with six, skinny, vertical squiggles.

3 Add seven curves on double lines...

4 and seven curls.

5 Finish decorating the cake...

6 and say "~~I do~~" *I won't!*

CALORIES EATEN:

appetizer + main + dessert + drinks = total

Ham

EVERYTHING BAGEL = **220** CALORIES

1 Draw two stemless cherries.

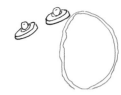

2 Put rings around them.

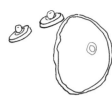

3 Draw two big wiggly ovals...

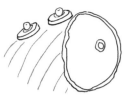

4 and two little wiggly ovals.

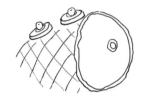

5 Draw seven curved lines in one direction...

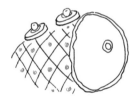

6 and six curved lines in the other direction.

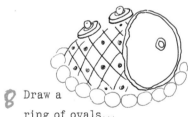

7 Add eleven tight little curlicues.

8 Draw a ring of ovals...

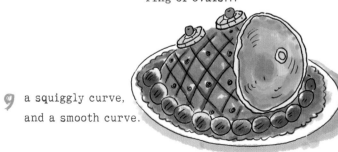

9 a squiggly curve, and a smooth curve.

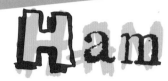

NO PORKING ANY TIME

CALORIES EATEN:

_____ + _____ + _____ + _____ = _____
appetizer + main + dessert + drinks = total

Lasagna

LASAGNA = **630** CALORIES

1 Draw seven pairs of curvy lines.

2 Connect the ends with curves.

3 Attach seven more pairs of curvy lines.

4 Connect the ends with curves.

5 Scribble in between the lines.

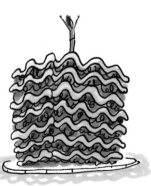

6 Climb high on seven layers of calories.

Tell your skinny friend she doesn't belong in our high fat club.

CALORIES EATEN:

_____ _____ _____ _____ _____

appetizer + main + dessert + drinks = total

Long Island Iced Tea

LONG ISLAND ICED TEA = **292** CALORIES

 1 Draw a cherry.

 2 Add a slice and...

3 a curve and...

 4 a zigzag and...

 5 an angle.

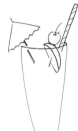 **6** Draw two toothpicks and a striped straw.

7 Attach two long vertical lines...

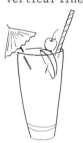 **8** and three horizontal curves.

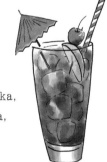 **9** Add ice, vodka, gin, tequila, and rum.

For a low cal alternative, skip everything except the iced T.

CALORIES EATEN:

_____ _____ _____ _____ _____

appetizer + main + dessert + drinks = total

Fat Potato and Skinny Potato

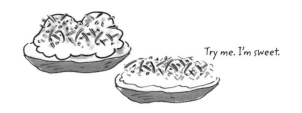

Try me. I'm sweet.

FAT POTATO = **900** CALORIES
SKINNY POTATO = **350** CALORIES

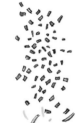

4 Top with bits of bacon.

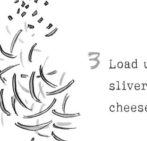

3 Load up with slivers of cheese.

2 Add two scoops of sour cream.

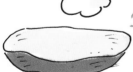

1 Start at the bottom. Draw half a potato like a lumpy boat.

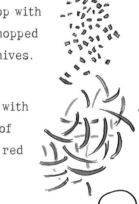

4 Top with chopped chives.

3 Load up with slivers of roasted red pepper.

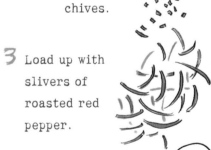

2 Add two scoops of plain yogurt.

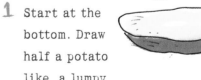

1 Start at the bottom. Draw half a potato like a lumpy boat.

CALORIES EATEN:

—————— —————— —————— —————— ——————
appetizer + main + dessert + drinks = total

Milkshake

MILKSHAKE = **914** CALORIES

1 Draw a cherry.

2 Add four squiggles on each side...

3 and three squiggles on the bottom.

4 Draw a double curve around the bottom...

5 and two lines angled down.

6 Attach a little loop...

7 a curve...

8 and a long, skinny, striped rectangle.

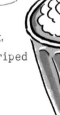

Why did the cow jump up and down?

Because she was making a milkshake.

appetizer + main + dessert + drinks = total

Margarita

MARGARITA = **168** CALORIES

1 Draw twelve roundish bits.

2 Put a line under them...

3 and attach two curves at either end.

4 Draw a bicycle wheel with spokes.

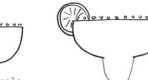

5 Attach a fat U on the bottom...

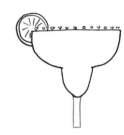

6 and a skinny square U on the bottom of that.

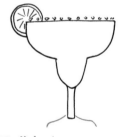

7 Make two curves...

8 and connect on the bottom. ¡Buenísimo!

CALORIES EATEN: _____

appetizer   +   main   +   dessert   +   drinks   =   total

Doughnuts

DOUGHNUT = **200** CALORIES

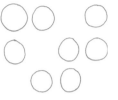

1 Draw eight circles in three rows.

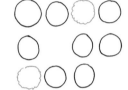

2 Add two squiggly circles and...

3 two really squiggly circles and...

4 six more circles and six more squiggly circles.

5 Fill in with 18 lines and a bunch of specks.

CALORIES EATEN:

_____ _____ _____ _____ _____
appetizer + main + dessert + drinks = total

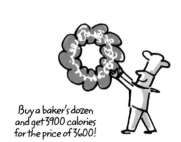

Buy a baker's dozen and get 3900 calories for the price of 3600!

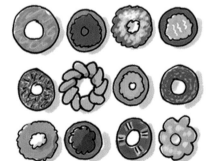

Cheeseburger

CHEESEBURGER = **350** CALORIES

1 Draw an oval...

2 and put 61 specks inside.

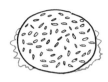

3 Add two squiggles...

4 two angles and two curves.

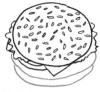

5 Put two more curves on the bottom...

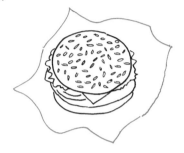

6 and a wavy line all around.

7 Order large fries and a soda for a happy calorie meal.

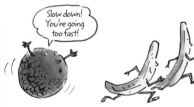

CALORIES EATEN:

_____   _____   _____   _____   _____
appetizer + main + dessert + drinks = total

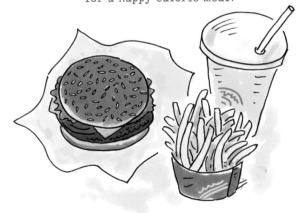

First and Last Bites

FIRST AND LAST BITES = **2,700** CALORIES

1 Draw two circles, four rounded squares, two squiggly circles, one rounded rectangle, one curlicue, and two round triangles.

2 Add three curlicues, three U's, four L's, six slices, one line, three blobs, 14 curves, and one dotted circle.

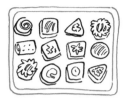

3 Put two rounded rectangles around everything.

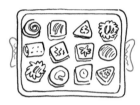

4 Add handles.

CALORIES EATEN:

_____ appetizer + _____ main + _____ dessert + _____ drinks = _____ total

I adore parties! You can have appetizers and dessert at the same time!

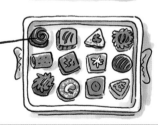

75 calories each

150 calories each

Filet mignon

FILET MIGNON = **580** CALORIES

1 Draw a scoop of butter.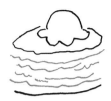

2 Put a slightly wiggly oval around it.

3 Add seven wiggly curved lines and...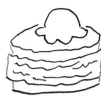

4 connect the ends.

5 Draw a blob of port wine reduction...

6 and slivers of green beans.

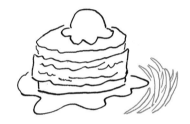

CALORIES EATEN:

_____ _____ _____ _____ _____

appetizer + main + dessert + drinks = total

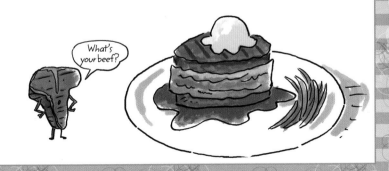

What's your beef?

Fried Chicken with mashed potatoes

FRIED CHICKEN = **850** CALORIES
MASHED POTATOES = **300** CALORIES

1 Draw a scoop.

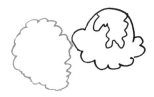 **2** Add a melted blob of butter.

 3 Draw a squiggly oval...

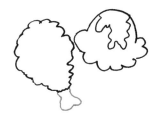 **4** and attach a squiggly blob.

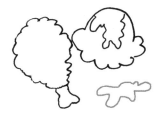 **5** Add another melted blob of butter...

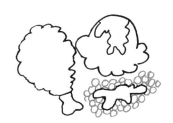 **6** and put peas under it.

CALORIES EATEN:

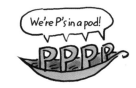 We're P's in a pod!
PPPP

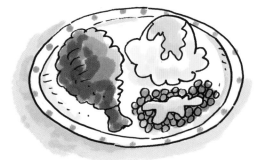

appetizer + main + dessert + drinks = total

Sundae

SUNDAE = **750** CALORIES

1 Draw a cherry.

2 Atttach one scoop...

3 two more scoops...

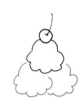

4 and just this once, three more scoops.

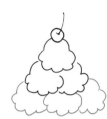

5 Draw two ultra curvy lines on the bottom.

6 Finish the dish with two lines, a loop, and a curve.

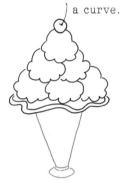

7 Pick your favorite flavors and...

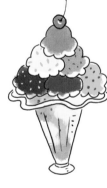

8 add sprinkles, syrup, nuts, and 8,000 calories!

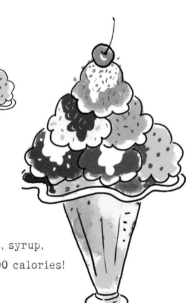

CALORIES EATEN:

_____ _____ _____ _____ _____

appetizer + main + dessert + drinks = total

Hot chocolate

HOT CHOCOLATE = **400** CALORIES

1 Draw a scoop of whipped cream.

2 Put a double oval around it.

3 Attach two lines down...

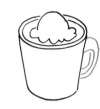

4 and connect with a curve.

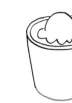

5 Add a three-curve handle...

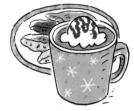

6 a matching plate of biscotti, squiggles of chocolate syrup...

7 and a cherry on top. Now put your feet up in front of the fire.

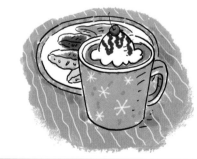

CALORIES EATEN:

_____   _____   _____   _____   _____
appetizer + main + dessert + drinks = total

Mudslide

MUDSLIDE = **441** CALORIES

1 Draw a cherry.

2 Add five curvy lines...

3 and a short horizontal line.

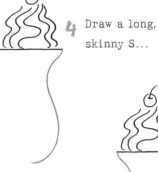

4 Draw a long, skinny S...

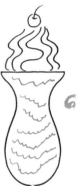

5 and a long, skinny, backward S.

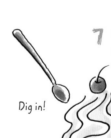

6 Fill your glass with seven wiggly lines.

7 Add a squared U and a curvy U and...

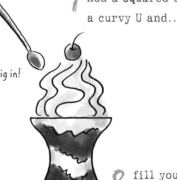

Dig in!

8 fill your glass with vodka, cream and coffee liqueurs, vanilla ice cream, and chocolate sauce.

CALORIES EATEN:

appetizer + main + dessert + drinks = total

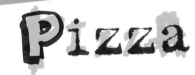

Pizza

1 SLICE WITH MEAT = **400** CALORIES
1 SLICE WITH VEGGIES = **300** CALORIES

1 Draw a squiggly circle.

2 Put another squiggly circle inside.

3 Add ten small circles...

4 twenty-five blobs...

5 and nineteen slices.

6 Cut your extra cheese, extra meat, extra pounds pizza into eight slices...

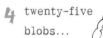

OR

6 savor an extra slice of veggie light-tomato pizza.

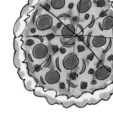

CALORIES EATEN:

_____ _____ _____ _____ _____
appetizer + main + dessert + drinks = total

Breakfast Bread

BRIOCHE = **280** CALORIES
MUFFIN = **100** CALORIES
CROISSANT = **280** CALORIES

1 Draw a scoop with five loops.

2 Attach six lines and connect the bottom with curves.

3 Butter up!

1 Draw a cloudlike blob.

2 Attach a squared U.

3 Add chocolate chips.

1 Draw a buttery curved rhomboid.

2 Attach two curvy V's on the ends.

3 Bake it flaky.

CALORIES EATEN:

_____ + _____ + _____ + _____ = _____
appetizer + main + dessert + drinks = total

Bread and Breadsticks

GARLIC BREAD = **320** CALORIES
BREADSTICK = **135** CALORIES

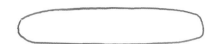

1 Draw an oblong oval.

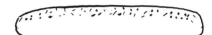

2 Speck it with garlic, salt, and herbs.

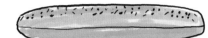

3 Slice it lengthways and slather the inside with butter and garlic.

1 Draw two parallel lines.

2 Connect the ends with curves.

3 Add salt and cheese.

CALORIES EATEN:

_____   _____   _____   _____   _____

appetizer + main + dessert + drinks = total

Carrot cake

CARROT CAKE = **415** CALORIES

  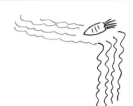 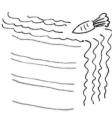 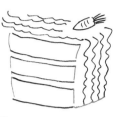

1 Start with a small carrot.

2 Add four squiggly vertical lines...

3 ...and four squiggly almost horizontal lines.

4 Draw six barely curved lines.

5 Connect the sides and bottom.

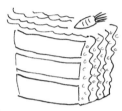

6 Add lots of little c's.

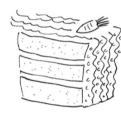

7 Tap lots of dots. The faster you do this, the more calories you will burn.

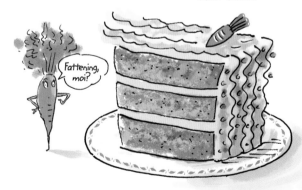

Fattening, moi?

8 Add a plate. The smaller the plate, the bigger your piece of cake will look.

CALORIES EATEN:

_____ _____ _____ _____ _____

appetizer + main + dessert + drinks = total

Broccoli cheddar soup

BROCCOLI CHEDDAR SOUP = **407** CALORIES

1 Draw seven squiggly blobs of broccoli.

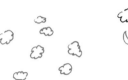

2 Add five slivers of cheese...

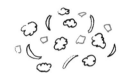

3 and five bits of bacon.

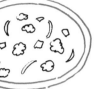

4 Draw two ovals around...

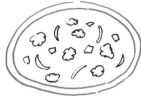

5 one curve inside and one curve outside.

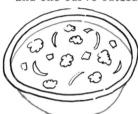

CALORIES EATEN:

_____ _____ _____ _____ _____

appetizer + main + dessert + drinks = total

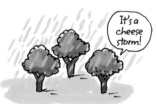

It's a cheese storm!

6 Dump in a load of cheese and a load of bacon while it's hot.

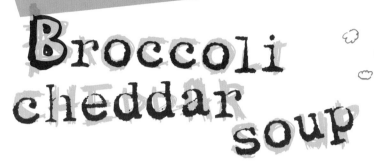

Manhattan

MANHATTAN = **210** CALORIES

1 Start with a cherry.

2 Add two straight lines on top and a curve on the bottom.

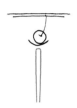

3 Draw a skinny loop.

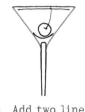

4 Add two lines...

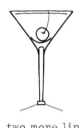

5 a little box...

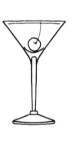

6 two more lines.

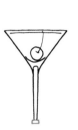

7 Attach a loop.

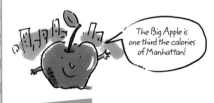

The Big Apple is one third the calories of Manhattan!

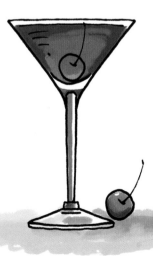

CALORIES EATEN:

_____ _____ _____ _____ _____
appetizer + main + dessert + drinks = total

Apple pie

APPLE PIE = **470** CALORIES

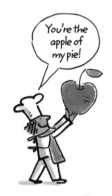

You're the apple of my pie!

1 Start with a big scoop of vanilla ice cream.

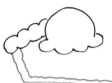

2 Attach a fat squiggle.

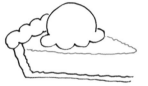

3 Draw two squiggly L-shaped lines...

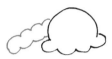

4 and one squiggly V-shaped line.

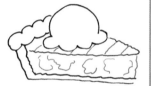

5 Add six short lines and six squiggles.

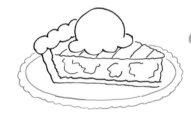

6 Put a smooth oval and a squiggly oval all around.

7 The pies have it.

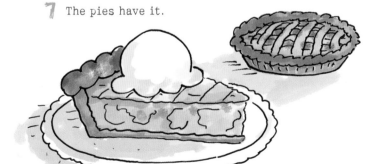

appetizer + main + dessert + drinks = total

French fries

FRENCH FRIES = **590** CALORIES

1 Draw a curvy V and I.

2 Make them fat.

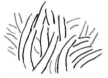
3 Add three pairs of curves...

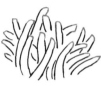
4 and five more pairs of curves...

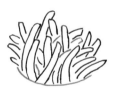
5 and nine more pairs of curves.

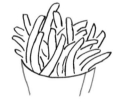
6 Close the top ends of each pair.

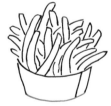
7 Draw one big curve and four small curves.

8 Attach three vertical lines . . .

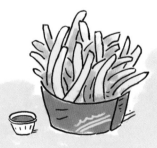
9 and connect with a big curve.

10 And get some catsup.

Cherry cheesecake

CHERRY CHEESECAKE = **450** CALORIES

1 Draw eight stemless cherries in a row.

2 Add seven small curves above and...

3 a squiggly line below.

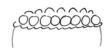

4 Draw two vertical curves on either end...

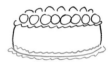

5 and three horizontal curves.

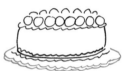

6 Add two more squiggles on the bottom...

7 and two vertical curves on the bottom.

8 Finish with two more squiggles.

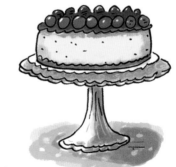

CALORIES EATEN:

_____ _____ _____ _____ _____

appetizer + main + dessert + drinks = total

Everything bagel

EVERYTHING BAGEL = **780** CALORIES

1 Draw two smiling bagel curves.

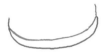

2 Slather on a squiggly curve of cream cheese...

3 and spread it.

4 Add a really squiggly curve of lox..

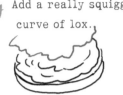

5 Draw two smooth curves and four u's of tomato.

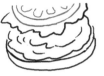

6 Add a really, really squiggly curve of lettuce...

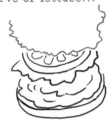

7 and three slivers of red onion.

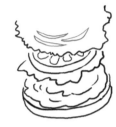

8 Put on the bagel top...

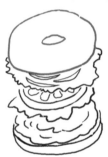

9 and everything on top of that.

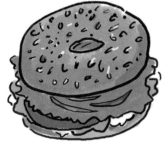

10 Carefully press down so that all of the calories ooze out the sides.

CALORIES EATEN:

appetizer + main + dessert + drinks = total

Wedding cake

WEDDING CAKE = **347** CALORIES

1 Start with six, fat, horizontal squiggles.

2 Connect them with six, skinny, vertical squiggles.

3 Add seven curves on double lines...

4 and seven curls.

5 Finish decorating the cake...

6 and say "I do" I won't!

CALORIES EATEN:

appetizer + main + dessert + drinks = total

Ham

EVERYTHING BAGEL = **220** CALORIES

1 Draw two stemless cherries.

2 Put rings around them.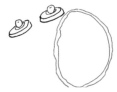

3 Draw two big wiggly ovals...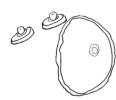

4 and two little wiggly ovals.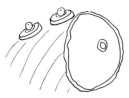

5 Draw seven curved lines in one direction...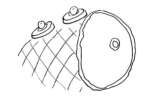

6 and six curved lines in the other direction.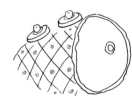

7 Add eleven tight little curlicues.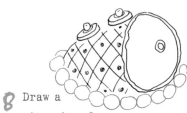

8 Draw a ring of ovals...

9 a squiggly curve, and a smooth curve.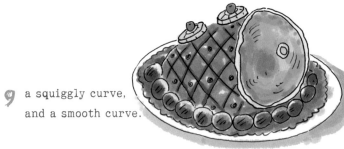

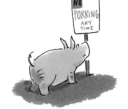

CALORIES EATEN:

appetizer + main + dessert + drinks = total

Lasagna

LASAGNA = **630** CALORIES

1 Draw seven pairs of curvy lines.

2 Connect the ends with curves.

3 Attach seven more pairs of curvy lines.

4 Connect the ends with curves.

5 Scribble in between the lines.

Tell your skinny friend she doesn't belong in our high fat club.

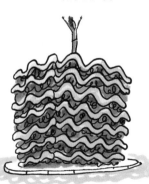

6 Climb high on seven layers of calories.

CALORIES EATEN:

_____ _____ _____ _____ _____

appetizer + main + dessert + drinks = total

Long Island Iced Tea

LONG ISLAND ICED TEA = **292** CALORIES

1 Draw a cherry.

2 Add a slice and...

3 a curve and...

4 a zigzag and...

5 an angle.

6 Draw two toothpicks and a striped straw.

7 Attach two long vertical lines...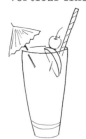

8 and three horizontal curves.

9 Add ice, vodka, gin, tequila, and rum.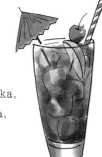

 For a low cal alternative, skip everything except the iced T.

CALORIES EATEN:

_____   _____   _____   _____   _____

appetizer + main + dessert + drinks = total

Fat Potato
and
Skinny Potato

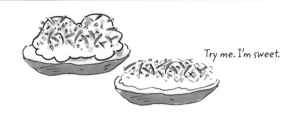

Try me. I'm sweet.

FAT POTATO = **900** CALORIES
SKINNY POTATO = **350** CALORIES

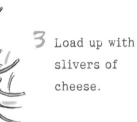

4 Top with bits of bacon.

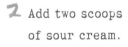

3 Load up with slivers of cheese.

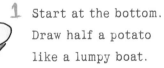

2 Add two scoops of sour cream.

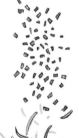

1 Start at the bottom. Draw half a potato like a lumpy boat.

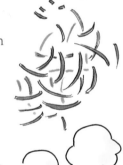

4 Top with chopped chives.

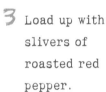

3 Load up with slivers of roasted red pepper.

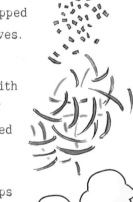

2 Add two scoops of plain yogurt.

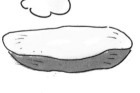

1 Start at the bottom. Draw half a potato like a lumpy boat.

CALORIES EATEN:

_____ _____ _____ _____ _____
appetizer + main + dessert + drinks = total

Milkshake

MILKSHAKE = **914** CALORIES

1 Draw a cherry.

2 Add four squiggles on each side...

3 and three squiggles on the bottom.

4 Draw a double curve around the bottom...

5 and two lines angled down.

6 Attach a little loop...

7 a curve...

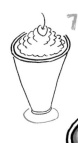

8 and a long, skinny, striped rectangle.

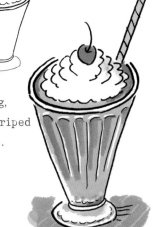

Why did the cow jump up and down?

Because she was making a milkshake.

CALORIES EATEN:

_____ + _____ + _____ + _____ = _____

appetizer + main + dessert + drinks = total

Margarita

MARGARITA = **168** CALORIES

1 Draw twelve roundish bits.

2 Put a line under them...

3 and attach two curves at either end.

4 Draw a bicycle wheel with spokes.

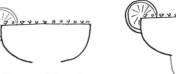

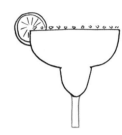

5 Attach a fat U on the bottom...

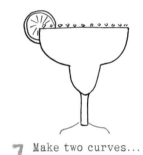

6 and a skinny square U on the bottom of that.

7 Make two curves...

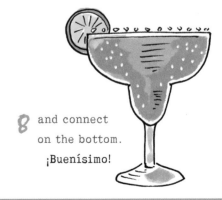

8 and connect on the bottom. ¡Buenísimo!

CALORIES EATEN:

_____ _____ _____ _____ _____

appetizer + main + dessert + drinks = total

Doughnuts

DOUGHNUT = **200** CALORIES

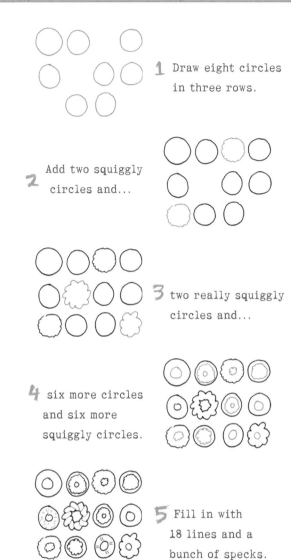

1 Draw eight circles in three rows.

2 Add two squiggly circles and...

3 two really squiggly circles and...

4 six more circles and six more squiggly circles.

5 Fill in with 18 lines and a bunch of specks.

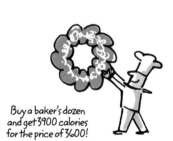

Buy a baker's dozen and get 3900 calories for the price of 3600!

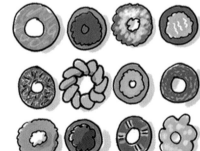